I0697643

DEDICATION

I dedicate this book to my sister who is fond of all my work. I will always be here for you, every step of the in whatever endeavor that you may encounter.

Table of Contents

Publishers Notes 2

Dedication 3

Table of Contents 4

Chapter 1- Introduction to Aromatherapy 5

Chapter 2- Know the Basics of Aromatherapy 8

Chapter 3- Choose the Best Ingredients to use for Aromatherapy 11

Chapter 4- Hazardous Essential Oil Used in Aromatherapy 15

Chapter 5- Have Your Own Basic Essential Oil Kit for Aromatherapy 20

Chapter 6- Important Oil Properties in Aromatherapy 29

Chapter 7- Learn How to Properly Use Aromatherapy Effectively 36

Chapter 8- Medical Properties of Aromatherapy 43

Conclusion 49

About The Author 52

Aromatherapy & Essential Oils Guide: Becoming an Aromatherapy Expert

The Healing Art of Aromatherapy

By: Barbara Johnson

9781634289924

PUBLISHERS NOTES

Disclaimer – Speedy Publishing LLC

This publication is intended to provide helpful and informative material. It is not intended to diagnose, treat, cure, or prevent any health problem or condition, nor is intended to replace the advice of a physician. No action should be taken solely on the contents of this book. Always consult your physician or qualified health-care professional on any matters regarding your health and before adopting any suggestions in this book or drawing inferences from it.

The author and publisher specifically disclaim all responsibility for any liability, loss or risk, personal or otherwise, which is incurred as a consequence, directly or indirectly, from the use or application of any contents of this book.

Any and all product names referenced within this book are the trademarks of their respective owners. None of these owners have sponsored, authorized, endorsed, or approved this book.

Always read all information provided by the manufacturers' product labels before using their products. The author and publisher are not responsible for claims made by manufacturers.

This book was originally printed before 2014. This is an adapted reprint by Speedy Publishing LLC with newly updated content designed to help readers with much more accurate and timely information and data.

Speedy Publishing LLC

40 E Main Street, Newark, Delaware, 19711

Contact Us: 1-888-248-4521

Website: http://www.speedypublishing.co

REPRINTED Paperback Edition: ISBN: 9781634289924

Manufactured in the United States of America

Chapter 1 - Introduction to Aromatherapy

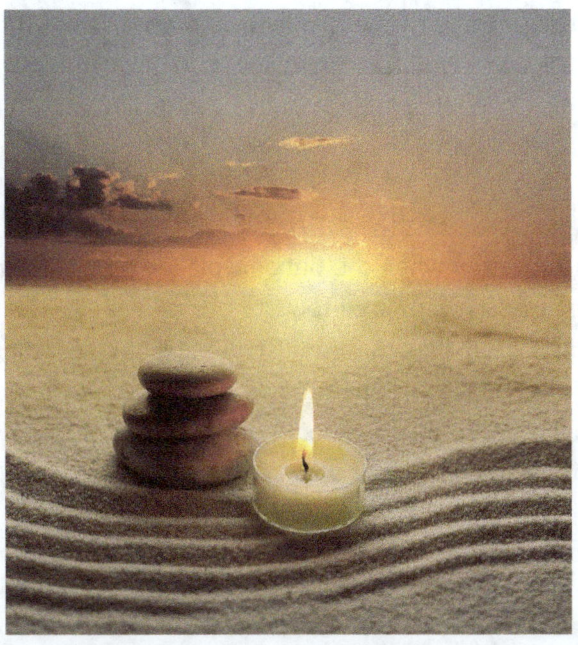

You have probably heard the term Aromatherapy and wondered what exactly that funny word, aromatherapy" actually means. It is the use of plant oils in their most essential form to promote both mental and physical well being. The use of the word aroma implies the process of inhaling the scents from these oils into your lungs for therapeutic benefit.

If you have ever used a vapor rub for a cough then you have tried aromatherapy, although not in its purest form. As a matter of fact, you probably have been using aromatherapy on yourself and your family for many years without realizing it through vapor rubs or electric vaporizers.

Vicks or other brands of vapor rub use eucalyptus or menthol to clear out stuffy chests and noses. Imagine if you used the undiluted essential oil of eucalyptus how clear your lungs would feel.

The term aromatherapy is generally new, beginning to be used in the 20th century, but the practice has been around for thousands of years. It is believed that the Chinese were one of the first cultures to use the scents of plants to promote health through the burning of incense. Ancient Egyptians used distilled cedar wood oil mixed with clove, cinnamon, nutmeg, and myrrh to embalm the deceased. The Egyptians also used oils to perfume both men and women.

In the 14th century when the bubonic plague hit, killing thousands of people, aromas were used to ward off the deadly disease. There is even discussion that the popular nursery rhyme, "Ring around the Roses" refers to aromatherapy. The lines, "a pocket full of posies" allegedly refers to keeping the flower in ones pocket in an attempt to keep the illness away.

Moving forward through later centuries a growth in books about the use of oils in healing grew.

The Greek alchemist, Paracelsus, used the term "essence" and focused study on the use of plants for healing purposes.

While the use of essential oils for perfume continued to grow throughout the ages its" use for medicinal purposes waned slightly until around 1928. It was at that time that a French chemist named Rene-Maurice Gattefosse accidentally discovered the use of lavender essential oil to heal wounds.

The story is told that he burned his forearm and reflexively placed it in the closest liquid he saw, which was lavender essential oil. He was surprised to find that the burn healed rapidly and left no scar. It was then that he began using the term aromatherapy and wrote about the powers of essential oils.

Today, many people are trying to get back to nature. People have seen firsthand the dangerous effects of synthetic chemicals and processed medications.

The use of all natural essential oils for medicinal, cosmetic and therapy purposes continues to grow. Many people have found the results of using aromatherapy to be far greater then manmade medications and with far fewer negative side effects.

Aromatherapy can be used by itself or in conjunction with typical medical treatments. For example, you may use aromatherapy to ease pain after a surgical procedure. You still get the benefit of the surgery but do not have to take the powerful and often dangerous pain medications that a doctor prescribes.

The basis of aromatherapy is in its use of naturally garnered essential oils. These oils are usually extracted from plant material and other compounds. The flower based oils are usually for strongly aromatic users while the other sources of oils are mainly used for medicinal purposes. These oils are primarily extracted from flowers or delicate plant tissues which are already known for their various attributes.

Surprisingly even in the culinary field, such elements are now becoming popular, especially among those with a more discerning palate. It should be noted here that such elements have long been used over time as a more traditional source of nutrition and even flavor.

Chapter 2- Know the Basics of Aromatherapy

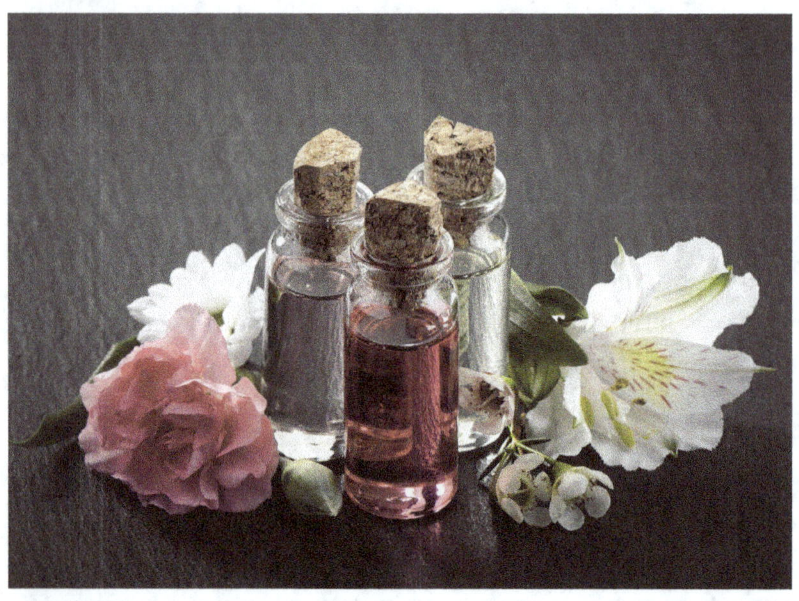

Most people today understand aromatherapy as just another indulgent exercise the privileged few enjoy. However upon taking the time to delve deeper, one is likely to find a whole new prospect relating to the very diverse uses of aromatherapy.

Aromatherapy can be explored as an alternative to more invasive methods of treatments. Originating long before medical science made discoveries and break-through; aromatherapy has had many success stories to back its many wondrous attributes. The concept of using aromatherapy to treat wounds and burns first came about when a scientist badly burned his hand while conducting an experiment and later it was used again successfully, as an antiseptic to treat the wounded soldiers during world war two.

Being the basis of natural materials, aromatherapy is less dangerous a method to choose from, when deciding on the best suited treatment for various illnesses. In theory aromatherapy is a treatment that may or may not help in the prevention of diseases by the use of essential oil. When coupled with the more conventional methods of treatments it has been found to produce impressive results, mainly contributing as a calming ingredient to the equation.

Aromatherapy can have a positive impact on the limbic system through the olfactory system. It has also been known to have direct pharmacologic effects. There have been studies done to prove the connection between the direct impacts of use between aromatherapy coupled with other scientific methods, however to date no conclusive data has been forth coming.

Sometimes divided into three distinctive areas of uses, aromatherapy has proven an effective solution to many problems. Aerial diffusion falls in the category for environmental fragrance or disinfection.

Direct inhalation is encouraged to arrest various respiratory problems like respiratory disinfection, congestion, tightness in the chest cavity and many others. Topical applications are mainly for relaxing purposes such as massages, baths, compresses and therapeutic skin care treatments.

Theoretically aromatherapy has been encouraged to be looked upon as an alternative to more invasive type of treatments. Besides being much more pleasant as a treatment option it can sometimes even be touted as a prevention element to certain diseases.

At worst it can play a major role in relaxing the general state of an individual and perhaps contribute in some way to the more successful percentage of recovery when combined with other more scientifically accepted methods of treatment.

Today there are many avenues of treatment to explore before embarking on a particular type suitable for the individual. However it must always be noted that before making a choice, one must always try to be as well informed as possible.

CHAPTER 3- CHOOSE THE BEST INGREDIENTS TO USE FOR AROMATHERAPY

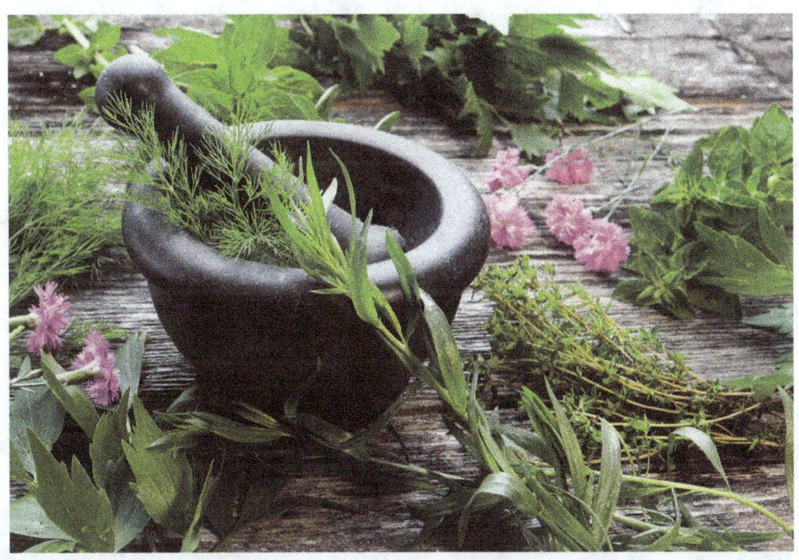

The general perception of aromatherapy is, getting the scent of an essential oil to infuse itself into the atmosphere to create a pleasing and relaxing state of body and mind. To others is may be perceived as a relaxing massage session with the use of beneficial essential oils. Using aromatherapy as a skin care regimen is also very popular.

Many of the essential oils used have proven qualities that can contribute to the various needs addressed in skin care lines.

These requirements can range from wanting to keep the skin looking young and supple to actually reversing the aging effects on the skin. Some forms of eczema and acne have been successfully arrested with the use of the aromatherapy method.

Aromatherapy & Essential Oils Guide

Aromatherapy is also an excellent way recommended to get oneself into a meditative state. These meditative states are usually associated with yoga, tai chi, visualization or self hypnosis.

Trying various oils before deciding on the one that best allows you to reach the required level of mediation is sometimes needed. Besides this some research has shown that using aromatherapy can help create the mood for various scenarios with specific results in mind.

Though there is lack of conclusive evidence to show aromatherapy can be instrumental in treating certain diseases, the fact remains that many people turn to this alternative based on other success stories.

Traditionally linked to the successful treatment of emotional and physical ailments there is proven success because aromatherapy is a natural method that helps the body cope with stress, anxiety and tension which are all contributing factors or causes of other illnesses and diseases.

Quality and Safety Control

Essential oils that are used in aromatherapy are not always easy to find. The Food and Drug Administration does not regulate essential oils so you, the consumer, will have to carefully read the ingredients of any oil you purchase to make sure that it is in its purest form.

In order to get the most benefit from aromatherapy, oils in their purest form should be used.

Finding the Best Essential Oils

Try to avoid synthetic oils. Essential oils are the only way to get therapeutic benefit from aromatherapy. They will not be cheap nor should many different kinds of oils be priced the same as the process of distilling them is varied.

Light exposure decreases the ability of an essential oil to work, so only buy oils that are sold in dark bottles. The term "oil" is often a misnomer as many of them are not at all oily. To test how distilled an oil is try dropping it on a piece of paper to see if it dissolves quickly and does not leave an oil spot.

If you have a health store in your area shop there instead of a perfume store. It is more likely that they will have real essential oils for sale.

Safety when using Essential Oils

Essential oils are very powerful when they are not diluted. In order to make them safe you should dilute them with carrier oil. Ask at your local health store which carrier oils they have available as there are many from which to choose. Follow the instructions carefully when making any essential oil compound.

• If a recipe says one drop, use only one drop. Anyone who has a nut allergy should also avoid carrier oils derived from nuts.

• Oils should be stored out of children's reach if accidental ingestion occurs contact poison control immediately. Pregnant women should consult their physician before partaking in any kind of aromatherapy.

• If you plan to use aromatherapy on infants or the elderly it is recommended that you use lesser amounts of oil in your recipe. Check with your physician to ensure that it is safe to use on a particular age group.

• Some oils can be toxic if ingested even in small amounts. In general, unless specified for oral use, essential oils should not be ingested.

• Essential oils stored in a cool dry place, and tightly capped will last six to twelve months. It is important to keep as little oxygen in contact with the oils as possible, so you will want to store them in full bottles, stepping down the bottle size as needed.

• Essential oils should never be put on your skin in their undiluted form. They can irritate your skin quickly and cause a chain reaction that will make you sensitive to that oil for a lifetime.

• Persons with asthma, epilepsy, or other serious health conditions should contact their physician before using aromatherapy.

• To avoid an allergic reaction, place a small amount of diluted oil on a patch of your skin. Cover the spot with a band aid and wait a full day to see if irritation occurs. This can avoid a potentially large allergic reaction to essential oils. Essential oils should be kept away from open flame or fire hazards as they are all flammable. Never use any sort of oil near your eyes. Wash your hands thoroughly after handling essential oils to avoid contact with eyes or mouth.

Chapter 4- Hazardous Essential Oil Used in Aromatherapy

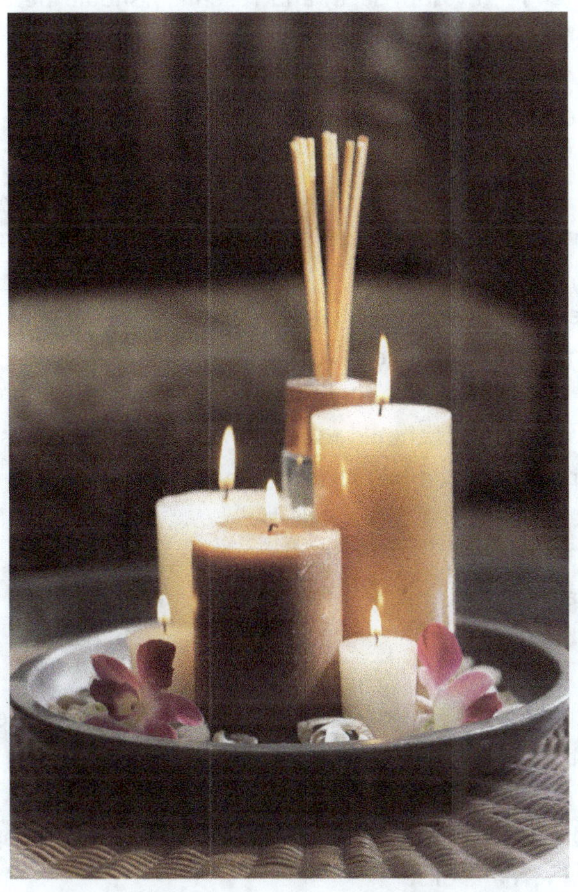

Hazardous Essential Oils

Some essential oils are very dangerous. These oils should not be sold at all, but can still be purchased over the internet or at less reputable shops. Others may be safe in some instances but can be rather dangerous if used in certain circumstances. Before you take on an aromatherapy plan, take time to understand which oils are safe. Keep in mind that just because something is all natural does not necessarily mean that it is not hazardous to your health.

• Rosemary, common sage, hyssop, and thyme should never be used if you have high blood pressure.

• Sweet fennel, hyssop, sage, and rosemary should be avoided if you have epilepsy.

• Diabetics should not use angelica.

• Those who suffer from hypoglycemia should stay away from Geranium

• Sufferers of kidney problems should be cautious if they use juniper, sandalwood, or coriander.

• Expectant mothers should especially avoid juniper, hyssop, clary sage, peppermint, lemon, fennel, lemon verbana, rosemary, and wintergreen.

• Clary sage should not be used while drinking as it will intensify the effects of the alcohol causing it to act like a narcotic.

• Chamomile and marjoram should not be used while driving because they cause drowsiness.

• Some oils can cause allergies, such as citronella, clary sage, ylang ylang, and verbana oils.

• Oils that are believed to be carcinogens are calamus and sassafras, should be avoided by everyone.

• Methyl salicyalte is the active ingredient in aspirin and sweet birch essential oil. If you use aspirin for medicinal purposes you should avoid it due to the risk of overdose. It should also be kept away from children as it smells sweet and is equally dangerous to them.

While the list above is oils that can be dangerous in certain situations there are other oils that should not be used in aromatherapy at all. These oils can be caustic if inhaled and should be avoided at all costs. This is not a comprehensive list, you should do research on any oil you plan to use before you purchase it.

Oils that should not be Used in Aromatherapy

• Almond - Contains cyanide which even in small amounts can be lethal.

• Aniseed - Skin irritant.

• Arnica - Can cause dizziness and heart irregularities

• Bergamot - Phototoxic, severe sunburn could occur if it is exposed to sunlight.

• Boldo Leaf - Produces convulsions even in small quantities.

• Calamus - Has carcinogenic (cancer causing) properties and can cause kidney and liver damage.

• Camphor - Oral ingestion can be toxic.

• Cassia - Skin and mucus membrane irritant.

• Cinnamon Bark - Skin irritant.

• Costus - Skin irritant.

• Elecampane - Classified as a serious skin irritant.

- Fennel - Can cause epileptic episodes.

- Horseradish - Eye, skin, nose, and mucus membrane irritant.

- Jaborandi Leaf - Oral toxin, skin irritant.

- Mustard - Skin and mucus membrane irritant.

- Spanish Origanum - Skin and mucus membrane irritant

- Dwarf Pine - Skin irritant.

- Brazilian Sassafras - Banned by the FDA as a carcinogen and can be toxic even in small amounts.

- Savin - Skin irritant.

- Southernwood - Toxic to the skin and if taken orally.

- Tansy - Can cause convulsions, vomiting, uterine bleeding, and death as a result of organ or respiratory failure.

- Cedarleaf Thuja

- Thuja Plicata - Can be a neurotoxin.

- Wintergreen - Can be a skin irritant, especially to those with aspirin sensitivity. The oil itself is poisonous.

- Wormseed - Toxic to the liver and kidneys, suppresses heart function.

- Wormwood - Consumption can cause visual and auditory

• Hallucinations and addiction. It can also cause convulsions and be a neurotoxin.

There are some essential oils that are highly toxic and should never be used in any circumstance.

Essentials to Completely Avoid

• Mug wart

• Pennyroyal

• Rue

• Sage

Chapter 5- Have Your Own Basic Essential Oil Kit for Aromatherapy

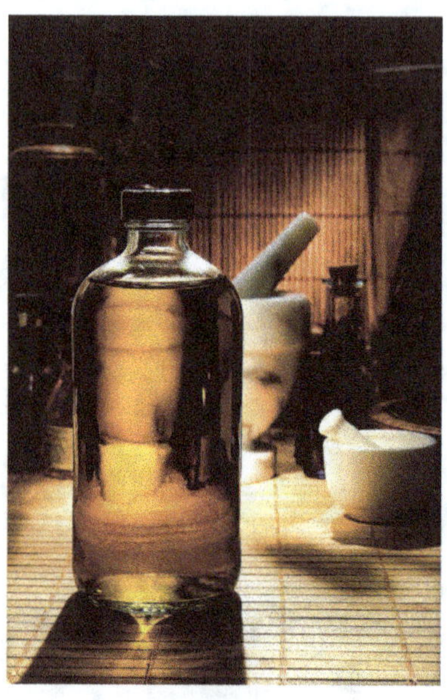

If you are just beginning your journey with essential oils and aromatherapy there is a few oils that will help you get started. These are some of the easiest to find yet versatile essential oils. Not only are they used for therapeutic purposes but can also be used in many other applications.

Some of these include making natural cleaning products and gardening. In addition to the oils you will need some way to get them into your lungs. An aroma diffuser is a good way to do this.

An aroma diffuser puts the essential oils into the air quickly and spreads them about the room which allows you to get your therapy by just relaxing and breathing deeply. They come in all different shapes and styles so you can purchase one that matches the décor in each room of your home.

Some run with the use of an open flame while others are powered by electricity. You can even get aromatherapy diffusers that work in your car.

Lavender

Lavender is a non toxic and non irritant essential oil. It is extracted through steam distillation from flowering tops of the lavender plant. Lavender has long been a folk remedy used to calm an upset stomach. Lavender has both soothing and reviving properties.

Lavender oil should be clear to pale yellow in will smell sweet with floral and woody undertones. It blends well with other floral and citrus essential oils.

As aromatherapy it has a variety of health benefits. It's pleasant and calming scent makes it helpful in treating nerves and headaches, anxiety, depression, and emotional stress. It also increases mental stamina and calms exhaustion.

Lavender essential oil is often recommended to treat insomnia as its scent can induce sleep. Massage with lavender oil can remedy all types of soreness and pain even when it is deep in the joints.

The vapor form of lavender oil is used to treat all sorts of respiratory problems including, colds, flu, chest congestions, whooping cough, sinus congestion, and asthma. Lavender has been used to promote good blood circulation and stimulate the production for gastric fluids to treat stomach ailments.

Tea Tree

Tea Tree essential oil is also a non toxic and non irritant but can cause sensitization in some people. This oil is extracted through steam distillation from the leaves and twigs of the Tea Tree.

Tea Tree has long been used by the aboriginal people in Australia and is named for their use of it as an herbal tea. The oil should be a pale-yellow green or water white color. Tea Tree blends well with lavender, clary sage, rosemary, and many spice oils.

Tea Tree oil is known for being anti bacterial, anti microbial, anti septic, and anti viral. In short, it can almost be called a cure-all because it has so many properties to ward off disease and germs. In Australia it is found in nearly every household because of these properties.

Tea tree oil can be used as an anti bacterial to cure all sorts of bacterial infections including the treatment of wounds. As aromatherapy it can be used to treat coughs, colds, congestion and bronchitis. It can also keep fungal infections at bay and even cure dermatitis and athlete's foot. Tea tree can be used as a stimulant to hormones and circulation and to boost ones immune system. Tea tree oil can help remove toxins by opening pores and promoting sweating which removes uric acid and excess salt and water from your body.

Peppermint

Peppermint essential oil is non toxic and when diluted is a not irritant. It can cause some skin irritation because of the menthol properties it holds and should be used with temperance.

The use of Peppermint has been seen as far back as Egyptian tombs from 1000 BC. It also has a history of use in China and Japan since the earliest times to treat all sorts of health anomalies.

Peppermint essential oil should be pale yellow or greenish in color. It has a strong grassy mint scent. Peppermint works well with other mint scents like eucalyptus as well as rosemary and lavender.

Peppermint has been studied in the science community and its health benefits proven. Because of this peppermint oil is available in pill form. It contains many minerals and nutrients like iron, magnesium, calcium, omega-3 fatty acids, and Vitamins A and C.

Peppermint is an excellent remedy for respiratory problems and is widely used as and expectorant to remove nasal and respiratory congestion. As an aromatherapy it can be used to treat nausea, headaches, depression, and stress. It has also been known to treat irritable bowel syndrome. As a skin care product peppermint oil can improve oily skin and replenish dull skin.

Chamomile

Chamomile is a non toxic and non irritant. It is extracted through steam distillation of the flowering chamomile plant. Chamomile has been used for over 2000 years in Europe for medicinal purposes. The oil should be a pale blue that will turn yellow as it ages. It will have a warm, fruity, sweet smell. Chamomile blends well with lavender and geranium as well as sage and jasmine.

Chamomile is well known for its calming properties. So much so that it can be used in aromatherapy to treat nervous disorders, headaches, and migraines. It is also used to calm allergies and asthma. Many women use it for the treatment of PMS or to relieve a teething or colicky baby.

Eucalyptus

Eucalyptus is relatively new to the aromatherapy family as it has only been used for the past few centuries. It is a non irritant but can be extremely toxic if ingested. It is colorless as an essential oil but has a distinct pine like scent. The essential oil is from the leaves of the evergreen eucalyptus tree that is native to Australia.

As an aromatherapy it is used to treat respiratory problems like sinusitis, nasal congestion, sore throat, runny nose, coughs, colds, and bronchitis. It is able to treat all of these ailments because it is antibacterial, anti fungal, and a natural decongestant.

Eucalyptus also has a cool and refreshing scent which makes it great for treating exhaustion and mental disorders.

Eucalyptus can also be used around the house as a room freshener, in making natural soaps, in saunas for its antiseptic properties, and even as in mouth wash or toothpaste.

Geranium

Geranium has many healing properties but can cause some sensitization and influence hormone secretions so it should not be used by expectant mothers. Geranium oil blends well with citronella, lavender, orange, lemon, and jasmine.

If used in aromatherapy Geranium oil is a great astringent. It promotes the tightening of muscles to keep skin from hanging loose. It has anti bacterial and anti microbial properties to help stave off infections of many kinds.

The essential oil is also known to be a cytophylactic which means it encourages cell growth. It can also be used to treat many mental disorders like depression, anxiety, anger, and pre menstrual syndrome.

Rosemary

Although Rosemary is considered non toxic and non irritant when diluted it should be avoided by epileptics, expectant mothers, and those who have high blood pressure.

The flowering tops of the Rosemary plant go through a steam distillation process to form the essential oil. It should be a clear or pale yellow liquid with a strong herb-mint scent. Rosemary is one of the first plants that were used for both food and medicine. In the middle ages it was used to protect against the plague and to drive out evil spirits.

When used in aromatherapy Rosemary oil can help to boost mental stamina and increase brain activity. It can also treat depression, mental strain, and forgetfulness. When one inhales Rosemary they will immediately feel uplifted making it excellent for relief of fatigue. It can also clear your respiratory tract and relieve sore throats, colds, and coughs.

Around your home Rosemary can be used as an air freshener and bath oil.

Thyme

Thyme essential oil is extracted by steam distillation from fresh or partially dry leaves and flowering tops of the Thyme plant. The oil should be red, brown or orange in color. It has a spicy and pungent odor. Thyme was one of the first plants used in Western herbal treatments mainly for respiratory and digestive health problems.

Thyme is anti bacterial, when used in its aromatic form it can prevent bacterial growth in and outside of your body. It is able to cure lung, larynx, and pharynx infections without effecting the rest of your organs like prescription cough medicines. Thyme is also know to boost memory and to treat depression.

Thyme essential oil is used as an insecticide both around the home and on your body. It can also help in treating bad breath and body odor.

Lemon

Lemon essential oil is non toxic but, it may cause skin irritation so it should be used with restraint. Lemon oil is phototoxic so exposure to sunlight is strongly discouraged. In Spain Lemon is known as a cure all-being used for everything from fever to arthritis.

The oil will be a pale green-yellow color that turns brown as it ages. It has a light citrus smell and blends well with fennel, lavender, sandalwood, and chamomile.

Lemon is very popular for cooking and for its fresh scent. As aromatherapy it can aid in the relief of stress, anxiety and fatigue.

The scent of lemon helps to increase concentration and alertness and bring an overall positive sense to those who inhale it. Lemon has also been used in treating coughs and colds and it the treatment of asthma.

The high amount of vitamins in Lemon oil makes it an immune system booster. It can also improve circulation and stimulate white bloods cells further aiding one's ability to fight disease. Lemon has also been used as an aid in weight loss.

As a household cleaner lemon can be used on metal surfaces like knives to disinfect them. It can also be used in soaps and facial cleansers as it has antiseptic properties.

Clove

Clove oil should be used with extreme care. It can cause mucus membrane irritation and severe skin irritation. As such it should only be used sparingly and well diluted.

The buds, leaves, stems, and stalks of the clove plant are distilled with water to extract the essential oil. It should a pale yellow color with a spicy scent.

Clove mixes well with sage, allspice, lavender, and rose. Clove has been used all over the world for centuries. It can be used to season food as well as for medicinal benefit. Clove contains many minerals including calcium, iron, potassium, and vitamins A and C.

Clove has many health benefits, namely in the form of dental care. It has germicidal properties that aid in relieving tooth aches, gum sores, and ulcers in the mouth. It can also help relieve a sore throat.

Clove is an aphrodisiac which makes it a great stress reliever when used as aromatherapy. It can also have a stimulating effect and help to ease fatigue. Clove can also be used to treat headaches, bronchitis, asthma, coughs, and colds. Expectant mothers can use clove to relieve the nausea and vomiting often experienced during pregnancy.

Clove cigarettes have long been a popular alternative to the traditional tobacco kind. At one time it was thought that adding clove could counteract the negative effects of smoking, this has since proved false. The American Cancer Society notes that there is no scientific proof that clove cures cancer in any way.

CHAPTER 6- IMPORTANT OIL PROPERTIES IN AROMATHERAPY

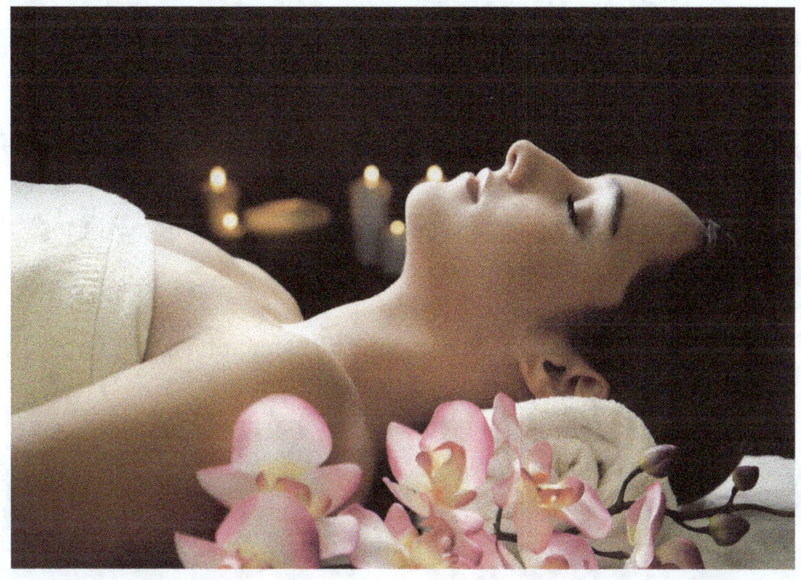

The properties of essential oils are what make them so beneficial. While most of them smell pleasant, that is just a byproduct of their real benefit. The term essential oil may sound simple, but they are actually complicated chemical compounds.

The ingredients in essential oils are organic because they consist of a molecule structure. This structure is made of carbon atoms and bound by hydrogen atoms.

In some essential oils there may also be oxygen, nitrogen, and sulphur atoms. By familiarizing yourself with the chemical make up of essential oils you can understand how they might benefit your health. In turn you will also be able to understand why some oils are hazardous.

Main Chemicals in Essential Oils

• Monoterpenes which have antiseptic and healing properties.

• Sesquiterpenes are anti inflammatory and anti infectious, they also have calming qualities.

• Phenols are a stimulant and best used in small quantities.

• Alcohols are antiseptic, antibacterial, antibiotic, and anti-fungal. They also stimulate ones immune system.

• Ethers are anti bacterial, anti spasmodic, and anti inflammatory.

• Ketones have relaxing and sedative properties. They are also an anti coagulant and can stimulate the immune system.

• Aldehydes can also be used as an anti inflammatory and to calm nerves.

• Coumarins are anti convulsant and anti coagulative. They can also be used as a sedative.

Home Recipes

Remember that essential oils are very strong so follow each recipe with great care. Less is more when making essential oil treatments.

Diffuser Mixtures

• For Attentiveness - 1 drop Cypress, 2 drops Cedar wood, 2 drops Lemon, 1 drop Pine.

• For Recharging - 2 drops Fennel, 3 drops Juniper, 3 drops Lemongrass.

• For Alertness - 2 drops Eucalyptus, 3 drops Rosemary, 3 drops Tangerine.

• For Motivation - 2 drops Basil, 4 drops Bergamot, 1 drop Clove, 2 drops Ginger.

• For Lucidity - 2 drops Bay, 3 drops Ginger, 2 drops Rosemary.

• For Calmness - 2 drops Chamomile, 3 drops Lavender, 2 drops Marjoram.

• For Harmony - 2 drops Benzoin, 2 drops Rose, 3 drops Verbena.

• For Peacefulness - 4 drops Bergamot, 2 drops Clary Sage, 3 drops Cypress.

• For Soothing - 2 drops Frankincense, 3 drops Melissa, 2 drops Patchouli.

• To Increase Socialization - 3 drops Litsea Cubeba, 3 drops Rosemary.

• To Relax - 3 drops Lavender, 1 drop Sandalwood.

• For the Kitchen - 1 drop basil, 3 drops Lemon, 2 drops Rosemary.

• For the Bathroom - 1 drop Basil, 3 drops Lemon, 2 drops Rosemary.

• For the Bedroom - 2 drops Bergamot, 3 drops Jasmine, 2 drops Ylang Ylang.

• For the Office - 2 drops Caraway, 3 drops Frankincense, 2 drops Ginger.

Bathroom Air Freshener Spray

• Fill a pump-spray bottle with 500ml of distilled water then add the following essential oils:

• 5 drops Cinnamon essential oil

• 5 drops Eucalyptus essential oil

• 5 drops Lemon essential oil

• 5 drops Sage essential oil

• 5 drops Thyme essential oil

• 10 drops Bergamot essential oil

• 10 drops Citronella essential oil

• 10 drops Lavender essential oil

• 10 drops Tea Tree essential oil

• Shake this mixture well before each use. Spray every day to keep your

• Bathroom smelling fresh and clean.

Lavender and Tea Tree Cleaner

• 1 t. borax

• 2 T. white vinegar

• 2 c. hot water

• 1/4 t. Lavender essential oil

• 3 drops Tea Tree essential oil

• Mix all ingredients together and stir until dry ingredients dissolve. Pour into spray bottle for long-term storage and use. Spray as needed on any surface except glass. Scrub and rinse with a clean damp, cloth.

Disinfectant Spray

• 3 drops Cinnamon Leaf

• 5 drops Pine Needle

• 2 drops Frankincense

• 10 drops Bergamot

• 1/8 t. Sunshine Concentrate

• 30 ounces water

• Combine essential oils with Sunshine Concentrate and water in a 32 oz. trigger spray bottle. Spray on and wipe surface dry. Disinfects countertops, stovetops and tile

Microwave Cleaner

• 1/4 cup baking soda

• 1 teaspoon vinegar

• 6 drops lemon essential oil

• Instructions: Mix ingredients to make a paste. Apply to interior of microwave with a sponge. Rinse and leave door open to dry for 15 minutes.

• Wash the glass turntable by hand. This recipe will get rid of food odors.

Floor Cleaner

• 1/4 cup white vinegar to a bucket of water

• 10 drops lemon oil

• 4 drops oregano oil

• Basic Wood Cleaning Formula

• 1/4 cup white distilled vinegar

• 1/4 cup water

• 1/2 teaspoon liquid castile soap

• 5 drops jojoba or olive oil

• Combine the ingredients in a bowl. Saturate a sponge and squeeze out the excess. Wash surfaces of tired and dirty wood. The vinegar smell will dissipate soon. Dry with a soft cloth.

Creamy Soft Scrub

• 2 cups baking soda

• ½ cup liquid castile soap

• 4 teaspoons vegetable glycerin (acts as a preservative)

• 5 drops antibacterial essential oil such as lavender, tea tree, or rosemary

• For exceptionally tough jobs spray with vinegar first—full strength or diluted, scented—let sit and follow with scrub.

Chapter 7- Learn How to Properly Use Aromatherapy Effectively

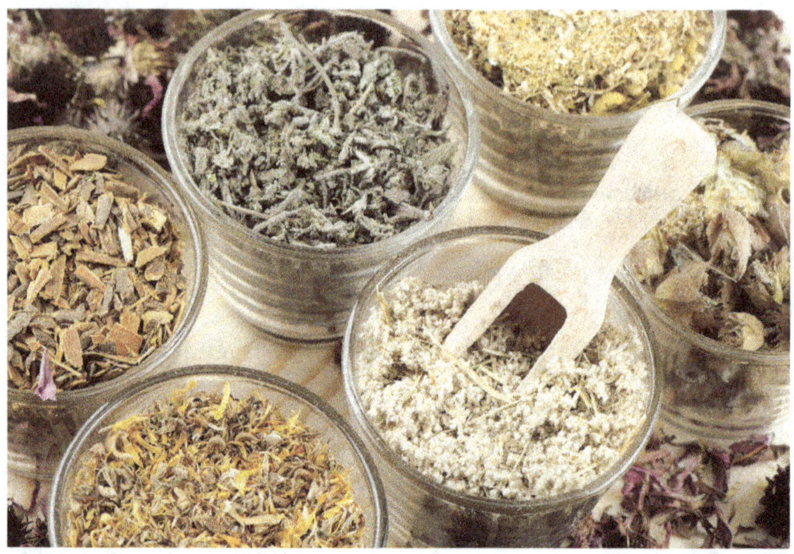

If one is thinking of setting up an aromatherapy centre or even considering the use of aromatherapy to treat a certain medical condition, the buying of the essential oils is a crucial aspect to consider.

Most essential oils today are so commercialized that it may not always be as genuine as stated on the labels. Careful examination of the label contents needs to be checked and rechecked before a purchase is made.

Some labels can be quite deceiving in their purported capabilities. The condition and type of packing of the essential oils is also a very important feature that should be considered. Ideally there should not be any cracks or broken seals as this will contribute to the contamination of the purity levels of the oils.

Besides all this, the other important fact to consider is getting the best results through the method and choice of essential oils.

Meaning some essential oil work better when used the correct way and the best results are assured if the recommended way is not taken for granted but adhered to carefully.

The method of inhalation is used to treat certain ailments like sinuses, headaches, colds, chest congestions and other similar conditions. This method is far more effective and quicker than taking oral or direct application on the skin.

Spraying a mixture of essential oils and distilled water is another method used to create a calming and relaxing atmosphere. This method has proved to be beneficial when treating anxiety, depression, stress and other pressurizing conditions.

Some conditions call for direct applications. However as most aromatherapy massage session are performed with direct skin contact, the concentration of the essential oils needs to be considered before commencing. Reason being that these essential oils could cause an allergic reaction to the individual.

More Useful Ways of Aromatherapy

Commonly thought of as essential oils just for relaxing, therapeutic massage sessions, aromatherapy is fast gaining inroads into other areas. Some of which are forays into treating ailments and some medical conditions that have previous success rates from using aromatherapy methods.

For years some cultures have used aromatherapy to treat wound and scars effectively. Using essential oils that contain the Helichrysum ingredient has been proven to be beneficial when repairing damaged skin conditions.

Its strong anti-inflammatory and concentration of regenerative dike tones is what makes it a highly regarded compound in addressing damaged skin problems. The pleasing earthy aroma it emits is also therapeutic.

Other essential oils that are also known for their healing properties for skin conditions are lavender, sage and rosemary. Sage is particularly effective in healing old scars and stretch marks but should only be used is small amounts because of the Thujone content which can be toxic.

Using aromatherapy to treat wounds is also widely practiced. This is because of the antiseptic elements that certain essential oils contain. Tea tree essential oil is commonly used to treat wound until the wound is totally sealed, after which this oil is no longer needed.

Some aromatherapy treatments are also used when the desire for healthy, younger looking skin is sought. These essential oils are absorbed into the skin and in turn provide the skin with all the important nutrients needed for the healthy look and condition.

Aromatherapy is also used in other products besides skin care. Products such as bath salts, shower gels, shampoos, body lotions. This style of using aromatherapy is wonderful for creating the desired effects of sweet smelling and relaxing moods. Also aromatherapy in this form is mild and non-threatening as it is not in its purest form.

Aromatherapy can also assist in relieving impatience and irritability. Essential oils like lavender can have calming effects on the mental turmoil state and works by encouraging the senses to slow down and simulates peace.

Approaching a medical condition by exploring the possibility of using aromatherapy as a solution is definitely worth the effort. Approaching a medical condition by exploring the possibility of using aromatherapy as a solution is definitely worth the effort.

The aroma therapist would have to consider factors like an individual's medical history, emotional condition, general health and lifestyle before putting forth any recommendations. This is a holistic style approach to treating a medical condition.

Some of the other more interesting conditions that are successfully explored using the aromatherapy method are backaches, irritable bowel syndrome, headaches and depression, to name a few. A good percentage of these medical ailments can be due to stress. Thus by using methods to understand and locate the individual's stress causing source, the aroma therapist will be able to alleviate the medical condition in a more efficient manner. In some extreme cases, claims of total recovery have been documented.

Treating skin problems is another avenue where aromatherapy has been successfully used. Conditions such as dermatitis, acne, eczema, psoriasis, cellulite, varicose veins and stretch marks are just some of the conditions where the use of essential oils has either arrested the condition or eradicated it completely.

Some patients have used aromatherapy to combat depression, hysteria, lack of concentration and panic attacks. Having tried other medically accepted methods which sometimes have undesirable side effects, aromatherapy has become a welcome solution. Treating burns, bruises and sprains using aromatherapy essential oils to achieve surprisingly quick and effective results are also another option worth exploring.

Other areas where the use of aromatherapy is being successfully explored are asthma, bronchitis, flu, and muscular aches and pains. When making the choice to use aromatherapy as a possible treatment for any given condition, it is important to ensure that only a qualified aromatherapy practitioner is consulted and that all the essential oils used are of the highest quality.

Be Cautious in Using Aromatherapy

Aromatherapy is actually a serious foray to embark upon as it involves the use of pure essential oil and other natural ingredients that are considered safe to use only if done correctly. Not understanding the attributes and purity of aromatherapy, can lead to serious repercussion as not all natural and pure oils are safe for human use. Some essential oils can even be toxic in certain circumstance.

Pregnant women and lactating mothers should be weary when choosing to use aromatherapy. The strong scents can be harmful to babies as their senses and immune system are not fully developed yet. Also some scents can be off putting to the baby and this may affect the baby's sleep patterns and feeding schedules, thus causing health issues from the neo natal stage.

Though aromatherapy has calming effects, using some essential oils to sooth and relax a cancer patient may have adverse effects. A doctor's permission should always be sought before trying this form of therapy. Some of the essential oils may have negative reactions to the prescription drugs already taken by the patient.

The choice made to use aromatherapy as an alternative to other medical options, should only be done after extensive studies have been made on the advantages and disadvantages.

Although most illnesses and diseases are found to be the root cause of stress, anxiety and other pressurizing conditions, opting to treat the medical condition by using aromatherapy may produce minimal positive results to actually combating the disease or illness.

Overenthusiastic use or indulgence of aromatherapy can lead to serious problems, especially when medical advice has been ignored in making this choice. Some studies continually show little of no evidence in demonstrating efficacy against bacterial, fungal or viral infections, thus rendering it a poor alternative to medically proven alternatives.

In most countries around the world, the aromatherapy use is still related to the indulgent relaxing aspect. Hence there is no regulatory body that strictly governs the content and potency of each essential oil used for the aromatherapy session.

Undiluted essential oils used for aromatherapy can sometime cause skin irritations and discolorations. In cases where the natural product has been exposed to chemicals in their growing stage, such as pesticides, chemical allergies can have a negative effect upon application. In more severe cases the presence of estrogen like elements, have been found to negatively affect the delicate skin of children.

Some cultures take the aromatherapy influence to the extreme. Ingesting certain ingredients is widely practiced and sometimes causes severe irreparable damage. As some of the essential can be quite toxic when ingested, medical advice should always be sought before advocating such a choice.

As with any bioactive substances the method of aromatherapy, using essential oils, and while safe for the general public can still have adverse effects when used by pregnant or lactating women.

Some of the ingredients and methods used in a particular aromatherapy session may cause negative side effects when interaction with other more conventional medical elements are present. Adulterated oils used in some aromatherapy session can also pose problems depending on what substance used.

Other safety issue like the unsubstantiated claims made by those advocating aromatherapy as a proven alternative treatment can be misleading at best.

Chapter 8- Medical Properties of Aromatherapy

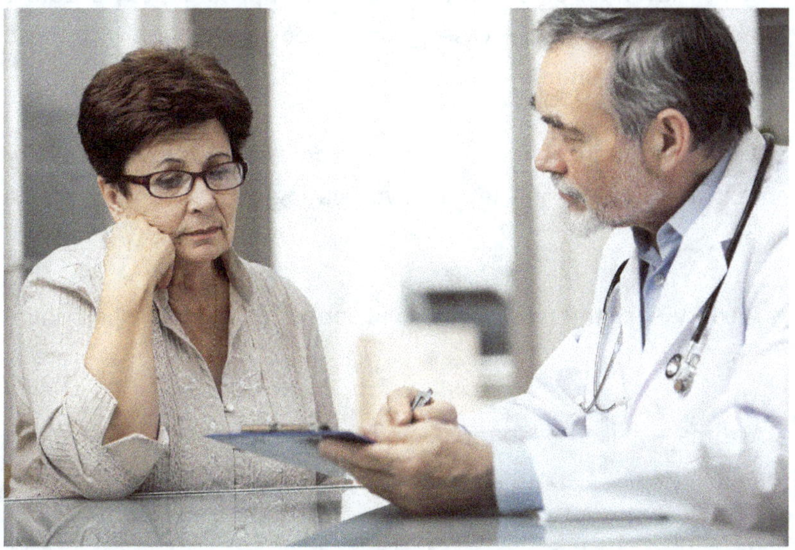

The popular belief that most illnesses and diseases are somehow linked to stress, anxiety and lack of proper daily nutrition has its merits.

Unfortunately some illnesses and diseases need to reach a critical stage before it becomes visible or is detected. To avoid all this, one is encouraged, though unrealistically, to keep all negative aspects in life under control or eliminate them altogether.

Wellness

Aromatherapy can helpfully contribute to this end. Primarily known for its calming properties, aromatherapy methods advocate the use of various essential oils to soothe the mind and body. Besides this a long list of other conditions can be successfully addressed with the use of aromatherapy elements.

Aromatherapy & Essential Oils Guide

Below are just a few examples of the capabilities and merits of using aromatherapy:

• Acne – lavender oil or tea tree oil to be applied directly onto the affected area. For milder cases, using a body bath lotion with these properties is recommended.

• Anemia – a concoction of tincture from the yellow dock root or an extract of dandelion leaf or even eating dandelion greens as a salad.

• Anxiety – chamomile, California poppy, passion flower, lemon Balm

• Asthma – ginkgo biloba, mullein oil, a Chinese herb called shuan huang lian

• Bee sting – urtica urens, cantharis, lavender and vegetable oil mixed

• Body odor – alfalfa contains chlorophyll.

• Bee sting – urtica urens , cantharis, lavender and vegetable oil mixed

• Body odor – alfalfa contains chlorophyll.

• Cold – eucalyptus oil in boiling water and inhaled. Gargle with a mixture of tea tree oil

• Cholesterol – chicory root, ginger

• Constipation – aloe vera juice, ginger tea

• Hair loss – saw palmetto, arnica, jojoba oil

• Headaches – chamomile relaxes, ginkgo biloba improves blood Circulation

• Dandruff – flaxseed oil, primrose oil or salmon oil. Rinsing hair in chaparral or thyme

• Diabetes – huckleberry, tea made from most beans

• Diarrhea – blackberry tea, wild oregano

• Eczema – chickweed added to bath, stinging nettle, hazel Ointment

• Indigestion – gentian root for better digestion, ginger, peppermint

• Nausea and vomiting – catnip leaves, chamomile flowers

• Menopause – for skin use geranium essential oil, orange blossom water, sandalwood essential oil

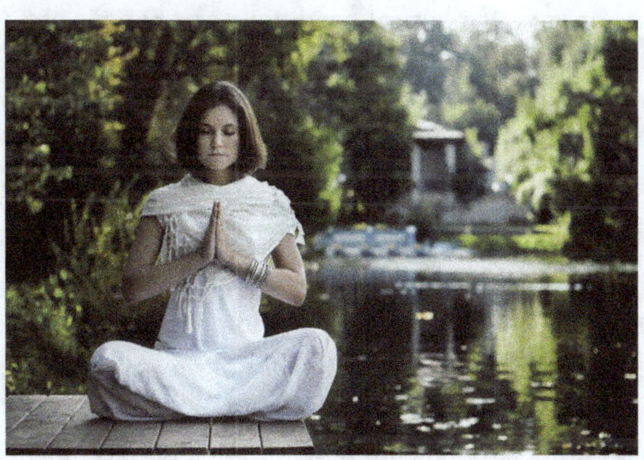

Digging More Useful Information About Healing Attributes of Aromatherapy

Confusing the attributes that come with using the term aromatherapy is mainly caused by the commercial sector seeking to capitalize in this area. For many people aromatherapy is usually linked to some pleasing scent emitted from essential oils.

The effectiveness in the aromatherapy element is in the application and intent. Aromatherapy is meant to create a positive change physically, emotionally, mentally or spiritually which is supposed to directly impact the body condition of the person undergoing a session.

However when products are touted to use or contain essential oils for aromatherapy purposes without actually comprising of the much needed dosage, it is no longer considered aromatherapy. Aromatherapy or commonly referred to as the practice of using essential oils for medicinal and therapeutic purposes covers Aromatherapy or commonly referred to as the practice of using essential oils for medicinal and therapeutic purposes covers many areas of healing properties. There are many essential oils used as remedies for various physical conditions and complaints. Essential oils are also believed to contain anti-viral, anti-fungal and anti-bacterial properties. There are also some essential oils that work well for various skin problems.

Don't purchase perfume oils thinking they're the same thing as essential oils. Perfume oils don't offer the healing benefits of essential oils. Even if you merely intend on using aromatherapy in your life for the out-and-out enjoyment of the aroma, essential oils that are breathed in may provide therapeutic advantages. These advantages don't happen with the utilization of perfume oils.

Don't purchase essential oils with rubber glass dropper tops.

Essential oils are really concentrated and will turn the rubber to a gum therefore ruining the oil.

Read as much as you are able to on Aromatherapy. It's really simple to get going with Aromatherapy, however there are safety concerns that you need to be aware of. You're wise to read even further on the significant subject of essential oil safety.

Be choosy of where you buy your essential oils. The quality varies widely from company to company. In addition, a few companies might falsely claim that their oils are pure when they aren't.

Learn to equate apples to apples if shopping for oils. Anise, lilac, bay laurel, cedar, and eucalyptus are examples of the basic names of plants utilized to make essential oils. There, however, are assorted varieties of each of these plants.

To differential these varieties, the botanical name is utilized to tell them apart. For example, two assorted oils are referred to as "bay laurel essential oil," yet they come from 2 assorted plants. The attributes and aroma of each oil do differ as does the basic cost between the two. It, consequently, is crucial to pay attention to the botanical name.

It's likewise helpful to note the native land for the oil. Most great essential oil sellers will promptly supply the botanical names and native land for the oils that they sell. When comparing one company's oils with another's, likewise pay attention to if the oils are organic, wild-crafted or ethically produced.

It's wise not to buy oils from vendors at street fairs, craft shows, or other limited-time events. A few vendors understand novices have no recourse against them later. This isn't to say that there are not extremely reputable sellers at these events; however this is a precaution for novices who aren't able to dependably gauge quality.

Buying oils from reputable mail-order companies might result in obtaining higher quality oils at lower expense than buying oils from a generic local health food place of business. Again, there's a wide variance in the quality of oils from company to company and store to store.

Store your oils in dark glass (amber or cobalt blue) and in a cool, dark place. Bare wooden boxes may be bought at craft stores. These boxes let me to move my oils from assorted areas of the house easily. Wooden diskette holders can likewise serve this purpose well.

Pay special care and attention to all safety data on all essential oils that you use. This is even more crucial if you have any medical condition or pregnant.

CONCLUSION

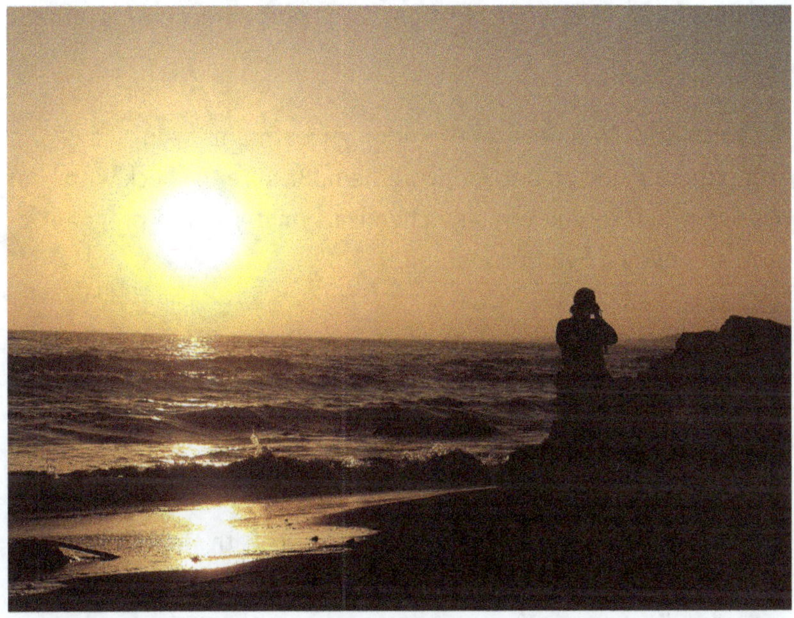

The use of essential oils can be beneficial to your health. These products in their natural form promote overall well being for those who use them. Instead of using complicated manmade chemicals, you use products what nature intended.

Not only can you maintain health but you can ward off illnesses like colds

and flu just by inhaling lovely scents in your home, car, or office. The use of essential oils will improve your health and raise your energy level.

Aromatherapy can even relieve tension and calm nerves. By using these complex organic compounds you can feel better and look better.

In addition to boosting your head to toe health the use of aromatherapy allows you to avoid using other dangerous products. When you use natures recipes to combat everything from diabetes to heart ailments you free yourself from the side effects of synthetic medications.

If you still require prescription treatment you can use aromatherapy in conjunction with them. Be sure to check with your physician before you mix any chemicals or if you are pregnant or have an ongoing health condition.

If you are just beginning your journey into the world of aromatherapy the kit listed here is a great way to get started. It provides you with commonly used oils that can be used in many recipes.

You should take time to familiarize yourself with the oils that can be hazardous especially as they pertain to your health issues or concerns. Remember that no two people are the same so what is a non irritant to another person may not be so for you. Simple tests can help you determine whether you will be allergic to an oil.

As a novice to the field of aromatherapy you should also take note of safety precautions and hazardous oils. Some less scrupulous sellers, especially online, will still sell things that you should not use in aromatherapy. If you see something that looks suspect trust your research and avoid it.

Once you experience the benefits of essential oils you will wonder how you ever lived without them. Soon your home will be free of manmade chemicals for cleaning and treating illnesses.

Do not underestimate the power of ridding your home of the scent of bleach and strong household cleaners. Imagine what taking those smells into your lungs does to your respiratory system. Now think of how it feels to breathe in fresh healthy air. This is what happens when you use essential oils to maintain a clean home. You and your whole family will be able to breathe easier and feel better. All of this by using natures essential oils through aromatherapy.

Aromatherapy is for you. It is meant to benefit your health and well being.

All the tools you need are some high quality, natural oils and a few recipes. More important is the knowledge that you do not have to do harm to yourself to keep your body and home free of germs, bacteria, and negative energy.

So, find a health food store and start stocking up on oils that you like. Smell them all and see which invigorates you. Build a beginner kit and start healing yourself with essential oils. Once you do that your only job is to breathe.

About the Author

Barbara Johnson is known internationally as an herbalist and aroma therapist. Johnson has taught seminars and other related workshop for over 30 years in different institution and organization.

Johnson believes the healing capabilities and other great benefits of aromatherapy. Thus, prompts her to create different books. She lives in Delaware with her loving family.

www.ingramcontent.com/pod-product-compliance
Lightning Source LLC
Chambersburg PA
CBHW070050260726
48658CB00002B/827